INTERMITTENT FASTING FOR WOMEN ABOVE 50

Unlocking Longevity and Vitality Through Intermittent Fasting.

Sandy D. Jakes

TABLE OF CONTENTS

Welcome to "Intermittent Fasting for Women Above 50: Unlocking Longevity and Vitality Through Intermittent Fasting." As I sit down to write this book, I can't help but reflect on the journey that brought me here.It all began with a simple realization - the feeling of sluggishness and a lack of vitality that seemed to accompany each passing year. Like many women in their fifties, I found myself grappling with the effects of aging, struggling to maintain my health and energy levelsOne day, a friend introduced me to the concept of intermittent fasting. Skeptical at first, I was hesitant to embrace yet another fad diet. However, as I delved deeper into the science behind intermittent fasting and witnessed its transformative effects firsthand, I became intrigued.I started experimenting with different fasting protocols, gradually incorporating them into my daily routine. To my amazement, I began to experience a newfound sense of vitality and well-being. The excess weight I had been carrying for years started to melt away, my energy levels soared, and I felt more vibrant and alive than I had in decades.But the benefits of intermittent fasting extended far beyond just physical health. I noticed improvements in my mental clarity, mood, and overall quality of life. Suddenly, the prospect of aging no longer seemed daunting - instead, it became an opportunity to thrive and embrace a new chapter of life with vigor and vitality.

Inspired by my own transformation, I embarked on a mission to share the power of intermittent fasting with women like me who are seeking to reclaim their health and vitality in their fifties and beyond. In this book, I'll guide you through the science behind intermittent fasting, share practical tips for implementing it into your daily life, and offer inspiration and encouragement every step of the way.

So if you're ready to unlock the secrets to longevity and vitality, join me on this journey. Together, we'll explore the wonders of intermittent fasting and discover the incredible potential it holds for transforming our lives. It's never too late to take control of your health and embrace a brighter, healthier future. Let's embark on this journey together - your best years are yet to come.

CHAPTER 1

THE SCIENCE BEHIND INTERMITTENT FASTING

Intermittent fasting perhaps you've heard the term thrown around in health circles or seen it touted as the latest trend in wellness. However, what is intermittent fasting actually, and how does it operate? In this chapter, we'll delve into the science behind intermittent fasting, exploring its mechanisms and shedding light on why it's gaining traction as a powerful tool for health and longevity.

My own journey into intermittent fasting began with a simple question: How can something as basic as changing when we eat have such profound effects on our bodies? It's a question that led me down a fascinating path of discovery , one that I'm excited to share with you.

WHAT IS INTERMITTENT FASTING?

Fundamentally, intermittent fasting involves alternating between eating and fasting intervals. Unlike traditional diets that focus on what you eat, intermittent fasting focuses on when you eat. By strategically timing your meals and incorporating periods of fasting into your routine, you can tap into a myriad of physiological changes that promote health and vitality.

You can also define Intermittent fasting as a pattern of eating that alternates between periods of fasting and eating, as opposed to being a diet in the traditional sense. There are several different methods of intermittent fasting, including the 16/8 method, where individuals fast for 16 hours and consume all their meals within an 8-hour window, and the 5:2 method, which involves eating normally for five days a week and restricting calorie intake on the remaining two days. Regardless of the specific approach, the underlying principle remains the same: alternating periods of eating and fasting.

Also, Intermittent fasting is a dietary strategy that involves cycling between periods of eating and fasting, where individuals abstain from consuming calories for extended periods, ranging from several hours to days. It's not just about what you eat, but also when you eat it, aiming to optimize metabolic health, promote cellular repair, and potentially extend lifespan by tapping into the body's natural rhythms and adaptive responses to food scarcity.

Intermittent fasting is a lifestyle approach that embraces the art of strategic timing in eating, orchestrating a harmonious dance between nourishment and abstention. It's a rhythmic cadence of feasting and fasting, sculpting a metabolic symphony within the body to unlock vitality, rejuvenate cellular mechanisms, and sculpt resilience against the ravages of time.

Let's break it down in a more simpler term

Intermittent fasting is like pressing pause on your eating clock—it's a way to give your body a breather from food, allowing it to clean up, reset, and recharge for better health and vitality.

Intermittent fasting is like a dietary rhythm, where you switch between periods of eating and not eating. It's a way of timing your meals to boost health and energy by giving your body a break from constant digestion.

Eating in cycles of times of eating and fasting is known as intermittent fasting. It's like taking breaks from food for certain periods of time, which can help with weight loss and improve overall health.

One of the key mechanisms behind intermittent fasting is its impact on insulin sensitivity. The pancreas secretes the hormone insulin, which is essential for controlling blood sugar levels and promoting the uptake of glucose into cells. When we eat, especially foods high in carbohydrates, our blood sugar levels rise, prompting the release of insulin to help shuttle glucose into our cells for energy.

However, constant exposure to high levels of insulin often driven by a diet high in processed foods and refined sugars can lead to insulin resistance, a condition where cells become less responsive to the effects of insulin. This, in turn, can increase the risk of type 2 diabetes and other metabolic disorders.

Intermittent fasting, by contrast, helps to improve insulin sensitivity by giving your body a break from constant food intake. During fasting periods, insulin levels drop, allowing cells to become more sensitive to its effects.

This not only helps to stabilize blood sugar levels but also promotes fat burning and weight loss which is a welcome benefit for many women over 50 who may struggle with weight management.

But the benefits of intermittent fasting extend far beyond improved insulin sensitivity. Fasting also triggers a process known as autophagy, which literally means "self-eating." It's a cellular cleaning mechanism that allows cells to break down and recycle damaged components, promoting cellular renewal and repair.

Think of autophagy as a housekeeping system for your cells. Just as you declutter and clean your home to keep it functioning optimally, autophagy helps to clear out cellular debris and maintain cellular health. This process becomes particularly important as we age, when our cells are exposed to oxidative stress and accumulated damage over time.

Intermittent fasting also activates pathways that enhance mitochondrial function the powerhouse of the cell responsible for producing energy. By ramping up mitochondrial activity, fasting helps to boost cellular energy production and improve overall metabolic function. This can translate into increased energy levels, improved cognitive function, and better physical performance benefits that are especially valuable as we age.

But perhaps one of the most intriguing aspects of intermittent fasting is its ability to induce changes at the genetic level. Research has shown that fasting can activate certain genes and pathways associated with longevity and disease resistance. One such pathway is the sirtuin pathway, which has been dubbed the "longevity pathway" for its role in promoting cellular resilience and longevity.

Sirtuins are a family of proteins that help to regulate various cellular processes, including

DNA repair, inflammation, and metabolism. By activating sirtuin pathways, intermittent fasting may help to enhance cellular defenses, protect against age-related diseases, and promote longevity a tantalizing prospect for anyone looking to age gracefully and healthily.

As I delved deeper into the science behind intermittent fasting, I was struck by its elegance and simplicity. Here was a strategy that tapped into the body's innate capacity for healing and regeneration, offering a holistic approach to health that went beyond simply counting calories or macronutrients.

But as compelling as the science may be, it's important to remember that intermittent fasting is not a one-size-fits-all solution. What works for one person may not work for another, and it's essential to listen to your body and adjust your approach accordingly.

In the next chapter, we'll explore the health benefits of intermittent fasting and how it can enhance cellular health and Longevity and also Mitigate Age-Related Diseases. But before we dive into the practical aspects, take a moment to reflect on the science we've covered in this chapter. Let it serve as a foundation for your journey into the world of intermittent fasting a journey filled with discovery, empowerment, and the potential for profound transformation.

Are you prepared to discover the mysteries of sporadic fasting and realize the complete potential of your body? Let's embark on this journey together.

CHAPTER 2

HEALTH BENEFITS OF INTERMITTENT FASTING

Intermittent fasting has gained popularity not just as a weight loss strategy, but also as a powerful tool for promoting overall health and well-being. In this chapter, we'll explore the myriad health benefits of intermittent fasting, from enhancing cellular health and longevity to mitigating age-related diseases. Drawing from my own experiences and the latest scientific research, we'll uncover how intermittent fasting can be a game-changer for women over 50 looking to optimize their health and vitality.

In a world where health trends come and go, intermittent fasting has emerged as a time-tested practice with profound benefits for both body and mind. In this chapter, we delve into the science behind intermittent fasting and explore how it can enhance cellular health, promote longevity, and mitigate age-related diseases. Drawing from personal experience and scientific research, we'll uncover the transformative power of fasting and its potential to revolutionize your health journey.

Understanding Intermittent Fasting

Intermittent fasting is not a diet in the traditional sense but rather an eating pattern that alternates between periods of fasting and eating. Unlike many restrictive diets, intermittent fasting doesn't focus on what you eat but rather when you eat. There are several popular methods of intermittent fasting, including the 16/8 method, the 5:2 diet, and alternate-day fasting.

Unlocking Cellular Health and Longevity

At the heart of intermittent fasting lies a fascinating phenomenon known as autophagy a process that holds the key to cellular rejuvenation and longevity. Autophagy, which literally means "self-eating," is a cellular cleaning mechanism that allows cells to break down and recycle damaged components. Think of it as a housekeeping system for your cells, ensuring that they remain healthy and functional.

My own journey into intermittent fasting revealed firsthand the transformative power of autophagy. As I embraced intermittent fasting, I noticed improvements in my energy levels, mental clarity, and overall vitality. Little did I know that these changes were driven in part by the activation of autophagy a natural process that kicks into high gear during fasting periods.

While autophagy is often lauded as a key mechanism, there are other compelling reasons why intermittent fasting is conducive to cellular rejuvenation and extended lifespan.

Enhanced Mitochondrial Function

Often referred to as the "powerhouse of the cell," mitochondria are essential for both cellular activity and the synthesis of energy. Through intermittent fasting, mitochondrial biogenesis is stimulated, leading to the creation of new mitochondria. This process enhances cellular energy production and improves overall mitochondrial function, bolstering cellular health and resilience.

Practical Tip: Incorporate intermittent fasting into your routine by extending your overnight fast. Aim for a fasting window of at least 12 to 16 hours, allowing your body ample time to undergo mitochondrial biogenesis and optimize energy metabolism.

Reduction of Oxidative Stress

Oxidative stress, caused by an imbalance between free radicals and antioxidants in the body, is a major contributor to cellular damage and aging. Intermittent fasting has been shown to mitigate oxidative stress by upregulating antioxidant defenses and reducing the production of damaging free radicals. By minimizing oxidative damage, intermittent fasting supports cellular longevity and overall health.

Practical Tip: Consume antioxidant-rich foods such as berries, leafy greens, and nuts during your eating window to further combat oxidative stress and support cellular health.

Activation of Cellular Repair Pathways

Intermittent fasting triggers the activation of various cellular repair pathways, including DNA repair and protein quality control mechanisms. These pathways are essential for maintaining genetic stability and ensuring proper protein function within cells. By promoting the repair and maintenance of cellular components, intermittent fasting helps to prevent the accumulation of damage and supports optimal cellular function.

Practical Tip: Prioritize nutrient-dense foods during your eating window, providing your body with the building blocks necessary for cellular repair and maintenance.

Regulation of Inflammation

Chronic inflammation is implicated in numerous age-related diseases, including cardiovascular disease, diabetes, and neurodegenerative disorders. Intermittent fasting exerts anti-inflammatory effects by modulating inflammatory pathways and reducing the secretion of pro-inflammatory cytokines. By dampening excessive inflammation, intermittent fasting supports cellular health and reduces the risk of age-related conditions.

Practical Tip: Incorporate anti-inflammatory foods such as fatty fish, turmeric, and olive oil into your diet to complement the anti-inflammatory effects of intermittent fasting.

Improved Cellular Stress Resistance.

Intermittent fasting induces a state of mild stress within cells, known as hormesis, which triggers adaptive responses that enhance cellular stress resistance. This phenomenon, known as hormetic preconditioning, primes cells to better withstand subsequent stressors, including oxidative stress and metabolic challenges. By bolstering cellular stress resistance, intermittent fasting confers greater resilience and promotes longevity.

Practical Tip: Pair intermittent fasting with regular exercise to amplify the hormetic response and further enhance cellular stress resistance.

Intermittent fasting offers a multifaceted approach to promoting cellular health and longevity beyond autophagy. By enhancing mitochondrial function, reducing oxidative stress, activating cellular repair pathways, regulating inflammation, and improving cellular stress resistance, intermittent fasting empowers individuals to optimize their cellular health and age gracefully. Incorporating intermittent fasting into your lifestyle, along with other healthy habits, can serve as a powerful tool for promoting longevity and vitality at the cellular level.

Mitigating Age-Related Diseases

Intermittent fasting has numerous advantages that go well beyond promoting cellular longevity and health. Recent research indicates that a variety of age-related illnesses, including diabetes, cardiovascular disease, and neurodegenerative disorders, may be lessened by intermittent fasting.

One of the key mechanisms through which intermittent fasting exerts its protective effects is by reducing inflammation a common denominator in many chronic diseases. By lowering levels of inflammatory markers such as C-reactive protein and interleukin-6, intermittent fasting helps to dial down chronic inflammation and support overall health.

Intermittent fasting also promotes metabolic health by improving insulin sensitivity and blood sugar regulation. As we age, our bodies become less efficient at metabolizing glucose, increasing the risk of insulin resistance and type 2 diabetes. Intermittent fasting helps to counteract these metabolic changes, allowing cells to become more sensitive to insulin and reducing the risk of diabetes and metabolic syndrome.

Moreover, intermittent fasting has been shown to enhance cardiovascular health by lowering blood pressure, improving lipid profiles, and reducing oxidative stress. By promoting fat burning and mobilizing stored energy, intermittent fasting helps to trim excess weight and reduce the burden on the cardiovascular system a critical factor in maintaining heart health as we age.

Harnessing the Power of Hormesis

But perhaps one of the most intriguing aspects of intermittent fasting is its ability to harness the power of hormesis a biological principle that states that exposure to mild stressors can trigger adaptive responses that enhance resilience and longevity.

Intermittent fasting, by imposing a temporary state of nutrient deprivation, activates a variety of cellular stress response pathways that bolster cellular defenses and promote resilience. These include the activation of heat shock proteins, upregulation of antioxidant enzymes, and induction of mitochondrial biogenesis.

In essence, intermittent fasting primes the body to better withstand future challenges, whether they be physical, metabolic, or environmental. It's a form of metabolic conditioning that strengthens the body's adaptive capacity and fortifies it against the ravages of aging and disease.

As I reflect on my own journey with intermittent fasting, I'm struck by the profound impact it has had on my health and well-being. From enhancing cellular health and longevity to mitigating age-related diseases, intermittent fasting holds immense promise as a holistic approach to health optimization.

But perhaps the most compelling aspect of intermittent fasting is its accessibility and adaptability. Unlike conventional medical interventions that often come with side effects and contraindications, intermittent fasting is a natural, time-tested strategy that harnesses the body's innate healing mechanisms.

As you embark on your own journey with intermittent fasting, I encourage you to approach it with an open mind and a spirit of curiosity. Listen to your body, pay attention to how it responds, and trust in its wisdom to guide you on the path to optimal health and vitality.

In the next chapter, we'll learn about adaptations and aging. But before we dive into the nuts and bolts, take a moment to reflect on the transformative power of intermittent fasting the power to unlock the full potential of your health and reclaim your vitality at any age.

CHAPTER 3

METABOLIC ADAPTATIONS AND AGING

As we journey through life, our bodies undergo a series of changes, some subtle, others more pronounced that shape our health and vitality as we age. In this chapter, we'll explore the metabolic adaptations that accompany the aging process and how intermittent fasting can influence metabolism in women over 50. Drawing from my own experiences and insights from scientific research, we'll unravel the mysteries of metabolism and discover how intermittent fasting can help optimize metabolic function for vibrant health and longevity.

Understanding Metabolic Changes with Age

As we age, our metabolism undergoes a series of changes that can impact our body composition, energy levels, and overall health. One of the most notable changes is a decline in metabolic rate, the rate at which our bodies convert food into energy. This decline is largely attributed to decreases in muscle mass, hormonal changes, and alterations in mitochondrial function.

Muscle mass, often referred to as our body's metabolic engine, plays a critical role in determining metabolic rate. Sarcopenia is the term for the process by which we age-related loss of muscle mass. This loss of muscle tissue not only reduces our overall calorie-burning capacity but also diminishes our ability to regulate blood sugar levels and metabolize nutrients effectively.

Hormonal changes also play a significant role in shaping metabolic function as we age. For women, menopause heralds a decline in estrogen levels, which can impact metabolism in various ways. Estrogen helps to regulate appetite, energy expenditure and fat distribution, and its decline can contribute to weight gain, insulin resistance, and metabolic dysfunction.

Moreover, mitochondrial function the energy-producing powerhouses within our cells declines with age, leading to reduced energy production and increased oxidative stress. Mitochondrial dysfunction has been implicated in a wide range of age-related diseases, including diabetes, cardiovascular disease, and neurodegenerative disorders.

The Influence of Intermittent Fasting on Metabolism

In the face of these metabolic changes, intermittent fasting emerges as a powerful tool for optimizing metabolic function and promoting metabolic health in women over 50. By strategically timing periods of eating and fasting, intermittent fasting can help mitigate the negative effects of aging on metabolism and promote metabolic flexibility.

One of the key ways intermittent fasting influences metabolism is by enhancing insulin sensitivity the ability of cells to respond to insulin and regulate blood sugar levels. Insulin resistance, a hallmark of metabolic dysfunction, is a common feature of aging and is closely linked to obesity, type 2 diabetes, and cardiovascular disease.

Intermittent fasting helps to improve insulin sensitivity by reducing insulin levels during fasting periods and promoting glucose uptake into cells. This, in turn, helps to stabilize blood sugar levels, prevent spikes in insulin secretion, and reduce the risk of insulin resistance and type 2 diabetes.

Moreover, intermittent fasting promotes fat burning and facilitates weight loss, a critical factor in improving metabolic health and reducing the risk of obesity-related complications. By extending the fasting window and tapping into stored fat for energy, intermittent fasting helps to trim excess weight and reduce visceral fat, the dangerous fat that accumulates around organs and contributes to metabolic dysfunction.

But perhaps one of the most intriguing aspects of intermittent fasting is its ability to stimulate mitochondrial biogenesis the process of generating new mitochondria. By subjecting cells to mild stress during fasting periods, intermittent fasting triggers adaptive responses that enhance mitochondrial function and promote cellular resilience

Mitochondrial biogenesis not only boosts energy production and metabolic efficiency but also helps to combat oxidative stress and mitigate age-related decline in mitochondrial function. This, in turn, can translate into increased energy levels, improved physical performance, and enhanced overall vitality a welcome benefit for women over 50 looking to maintain their zest for life.

As I reflect on my own journey with intermittent fasting, I'm struck by the profound impact it has had on my metabolic health and overall well-being. From improving insulin sensitivity and promoting fat loss to enhancing mitochondrial function and metabolic flexibility, intermittent fasting offers a holistic approach to optimizing metabolic health in women over 50.

But perhaps the most empowering aspect of intermittent fasting is its ability to harness the body's innate capacity for adaptation and resilience. By challenging our metabolic systems in a controlled manner, intermittent fasting primes the body to better withstand the rigors of aging and maintain metabolic health and vitality well into the golden years.

As you embark on your own journey with intermittent fasting, I encourage you to approach it with an open mind and a spirit of curiosity. Listen to your body, honor its signals, and trust in its ability to adapt and thrive in response to the challenges you encounter along the way.

In the next chapter, we'll talk about Hormonal regulations and Longevity and the impact of intermittent fasting on menopause and hormonal health.

Are you as excited as I am?

CHAPTER 4

HORMONAL REGULATIONS AND LONGEVITY

In the journey towards enhancing longevity and overall well-being, understanding hormonal regulation plays a pivotal role. Hormones act as messengers within the body, orchestrating various physiological processes, including growth, metabolism, reproduction, and stress response. Maintaining hormonal balance is crucial for optimal health and longevity.

Hormonal Regulation

1. The Endocrine System

The endocrine system comprises glands that produce hormones, such as the thyroid, adrenal glands, pancreas, and reproductive organs. These hormones travel through the bloodstream, affecting target tissues and organs.

2. Key Hormones

Insulin: Regulates blood sugar levels.

Thyroid Hormones: Control metabolism.

Cortisol: Regulates stress response.

Sex Hormones (Estrogen, Testosterone): Influence reproductive health and vitality.

3. Hormonal Imbalance

Hormonal imbalance can result from various factors, including stress, poor diet, lack of exercise, and aging. Imbalances may lead to symptoms such as fatigue, weight gain, mood swings, and decreased libido.

Balancing Hormones Through Intermittent Fasting

Intermittent fasting (IF) has gained popularity as a strategy for promoting hormonal balance and longevity. Here are practical tips for incorporating intermittent fasting into your routine:

1. **Start Gradually**

Begin with shorter fasting periods, such as 12-14 hours overnight, and gradually extend the fasting window as your body adjusts.

2. **Choose an IF Method**

There are several IF protocols, including the 16/8 method (fasting for 16 hours, eating within an 8-hour window), 5:2 method (eating normally for 5 days, restricting calories for 2 days), and alternate-day fasting. Experiment to find the method that suits your lifestyle best.

3. Stay Hydrated

Drink plenty of water during fasting periods to stay hydrated and support metabolic processes.

4. Focus on Nutrient-Dense Foods

During eating windows, prioritize whole, nutrient-dense foods such as fruits, vegetables, lean proteins, and healthy fats to support hormonal balance and overall health.

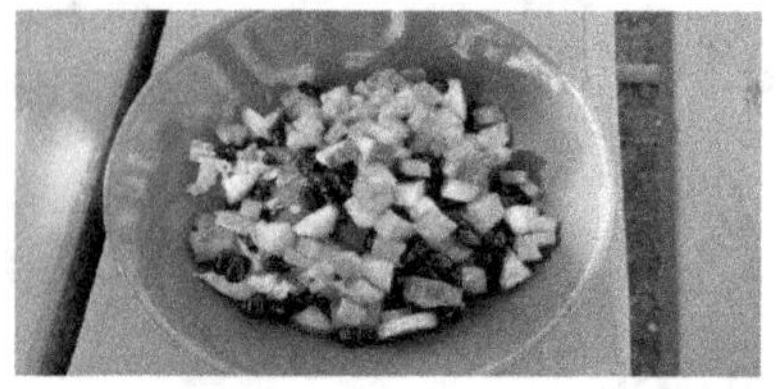

5. Monitor Energy Levels

Keep an eye on how fasting affects your body. If you experience excessive fatigue or other adverse effects, adjust your fasting schedule or consult a healthcare professional.

6. **Be Consistent**

The secret to enjoying the advantages of intermittent fasting is consistency. Stick to your fasting schedule to allow your body to adapt and optimize hormone regulation.

Impacts of Fasting on Menopause and Hormonal Health

Menopause, a natural transition marking the end of reproductive years in women, is characterized by hormonal changes, particularly a decline in estrogen levels. Intermittent fasting can potentially influence menopausal symptoms and hormonal health in the following ways:

1. **Weight Management:** Intermittent fasting may aid in weight management by promoting fat loss and improving metabolic health, which can be beneficial for women experiencing weight gain during menopause.

2. **Insulin Sensitivity:** Fasting has been shown to enhance insulin sensitivity, which may help mitigate insulin resistance and reduce the risk of type 2 diabetes, a concern for some menopausal women.

3. **Hormone Balance:**While research specifically on menopausal women and fasting is limited, intermittent fasting's potential to regulate insulin and other hormones suggests it may help alleviate menopausal symptoms such as hot flashes, mood swings, and sleep disturbances.

4. **Bone Health:** Adequate nutrition during eating windows is essential for maintaining bone health, especially during menopause when women are at increased risk of osteoporosis. Make sure you're getting enough calcium, vitamin D, and other nutrients that promote healthy bones..

5. **Consultation and Monitoring:** Women considering intermittent fasting during menopause should consult with a healthcare provider to ensure it aligns with their individual health needs and medical history. Regular monitoring of hormonal levels and overall health is recommended.

In conclusion, hormonal regulation plays a crucial role in longevity and overall health. Intermittent fasting offers a promising approach to support hormone balance and promote well-being. By adopting healthy lifestyle practices, including intermittent fasting, individuals can optimize hormonal

health and enhance longevity for a fulfilling
life.

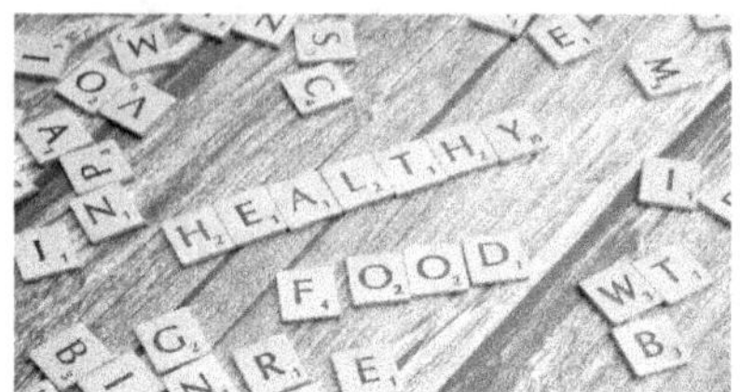

CHAPTER 5

CELLULAR REPAIR AND ANTI-AGING EFFECTS

In our quest for longevity and vitality, understanding the intricate mechanisms of cellular repair and anti-aging effects holds profound significance. This chapter delves into the fascinating realm of cellular repair, highlighting the pivotal role of autophagy, exploring the rejuvenating effects of fasting, and shedding light on the journey of aging women seeking cellular regeneration.

Exploring Autophagy: The Cellular Cleanup Crew

Imagine your cells as bustling cities, with intricate pathways and structures bustling with activity. Just as cities require maintenance to thrive, our cells too rely on mechanisms like autophagy for their upkeep. Autophagy, derived from the Greek words "auto" meaning self, and "phagy" meaning eat, is essentially the cellular process of self-cleaning and recycling.

Personal Insight: My Journey into Exploring Autophagy

Embarking on my journey into the realm of longevity, I stumbled upon the marvels of autophagy. Through fasting and mindful lifestyle choices, I sought to harness the innate potential of my cells for rejuvenation and repair.

Autophagy serves as the cellular clean up crew, identifying and removing damaged organelles, misfolded proteins, and other cellular debris. Think of it as a meticulous janitorial service, ensuring cellular health and functionality.

The Role of Autophagy in Longevity

As we age, our cells accumulate wear and tear, leading to a decline in function and vitality. Herein lies the significance of autophagy in promoting longevity. By clearing out cellular clutter, autophagy fosters a conducive environment for cellular repair and regeneration.

Consider the analogy of a cluttered attic: over time, the accumulation of unused items hampers functionality and diminishes the space's potential. Autophagy acts as the diligent organizer, decluttering the attic of our cells and restoring them to their optimal state.

Fasting: Igniting Cellular Regeneration

Fasting, long revered for its spiritual and therapeutic benefits, has emerged as a potent catalyst for cellular regeneration and anti-aging effects. By temporarily abstaining from food, fasting triggers a cascade of molecular pathways, including the upregulation of autophagy.

Personal Experience: Fasting and Cellular Rejuvenation in Aging Women

In my journey of self-discovery, fasting emerged as a transformative tool for cellular rejuvenation. As an aging woman, I embraced intermittent fasting not only as a dietary practice but as a profound means of nurturing my cells and defying the effects of time.

During fasting, the body switches from a state of growth and proliferation to one of repair and renewal. As nutrient availability dwindles, cells tap into their internal reserves, initiating autophagy to sustain vital functions and mitigate cellular damage.

Harnessing the Power of Nutrient Sensing Pathways

Central to the orchestration of cellular repair and anti-aging effects are nutrient sensing pathways such as mTOR (mechanistic target of rapamycin) and AMPK (AMP-activated protein kinase). These molecular switches govern cellular metabolism and play a pivotal role in modulating autophagy in response to nutrient availability.

Imagine mTOR as a traffic signal: when nutrients abound, mTOR signals cells to prioritize growth and proliferation. Conversely, during fasting or nutrient scarcity, mTOR activity wanes, paving the way for autophagy activation and cellular repair.

Lifestyle Strategies for Enhancing Cellular Repair

In our journey towards optimal health and longevity, adopting lifestyle strategies that promote cellular repair and anti-aging effects is paramount. Beyond fasting, incorporating nutrient-dense foods, regular exercise, stress management techniques, and adequate sleep are integral components of a holistic approach to cellular rejuvenation.

Personal Reflection: Nurturing the Temple Within

As I traverse the path of aging with grace and vitality, I am reminded of the profound interconnectedness between mind, body, and spirit. Through mindful lifestyle choices and a deep reverence for the innate wisdom of my cells, I strive to nurture the temple within and cultivate a harmonious environment conducive to cellular repair and longevity.

Embracing the Journey of Cellular Renewal

In the labyrinth of life, our cells serve as faithful companions, steadfast in their quest for equilibrium and renewal. Through the prism of autophagy, fasting, and lifestyle optimization, we glimpse the boundless potential for cellular repair and anti-aging effects.

As we traverse the ever-unfolding tapestry of existence, let us embrace the journey of cellular renewal with reverence and awe. For in the intricate dance of life, lies the eternal symphony of regeneration and vitality, beckoning us to embrace each moment with gratitude and resilience.

May we, as stewards of our own well-being, honor the sacred covenant between body, mind, and spirit, and embark upon the path of cellular rejuvenation with courage and grace.

The chapter encapsulates the intricate dance of cellular repair and anti-aging effects, weaving personal insights with scientific discourse to illuminate the transformative power of autophagy and fasting in the pursuit of longevity. Through mindful lifestyle choices and a deep reverence for the innate wisdom of our cells, we embark upon a journey of cellular renewal, guided by the timeless rhythm of regeneration and vitality.

CHAPTER 6

COGNITIVE HEALTH AND BRAIN AGING

In the tapestry of aging, preserving cognitive health and warding off the effects of brain aging stand as paramount concerns. This chapter illuminates the intricacies of cognitive health, delving into the nuances of brain aging while exploring the neuroprotective effects of intermittent fasting in aging women.

Understanding Cognitive Health

Cognitive health encompasses the intricate network of mental processes that enable us to perceive, comprehend, and navigate the world around us. From memory and attention to problem-solving and decision-making, cognitive function forms the bedrock of our daily existence.

As we age, however, the specter of cognitive decline looms large, encompassing a spectrum of changes ranging from mild forgetfulness to debilitating conditions like Alzheimer's disease and dementia.

Practical Tips for Fasting's Influence on Brain Function

Intermittent fasting, characterized by cycles of eating and fasting periods, has garnered attention for its potential to bolster brain function and mitigate cognitive decline. Here are practical tips to harness the neuroprotective effects of fasting:

Start Slow: Begin with shorter fasting windows, gradually extending fasting periods as your body adjusts. Aim for a fasting duration that feels sustainable and comfortable for you.

Stay Hydrated: During fasting periods, prioritize hydration by drinking plenty of water and herbal teas. Proper hydration supports cognitive function and helps stave off fatigue.

Mindful Eating: When breaking your fast, opt for nutrient-dense foods rich in antioxidants, omega-3 fatty acids, and brain-boosting nutrients. Make sure your meals are rich in fruits, veggies, lean proteins, and healthy fats.

Pay Attention to Your Body Recognize your body's hunger signs and heed them. If fasting feels overly challenging or triggers adverse effects, consider adjusting your approach or seeking guidance from a healthcare professional.

Neuroprotective Effects of Intermittent Fasting in Aging Women

For aging women, intermittent fasting holds promise as a potent ally in the fight against cognitive decline. Research suggests that fasting triggers molecular pathways that enhance brain plasticity, promote the production of neurotrophic factors, and mitigate neuroinflammation.

By fostering a brain-friendly environment characterized by enhanced neuronal resilience and adaptive stress responses, intermittent fasting empowers aging women to safeguard cognitive function and preserve brain health.

Embracing the Journey of Brain Aging

As we traverse the terrain of brain aging, let us embrace the journey with curiosity, resilience, and a commitment to holistic well-being. Beyond the realm of fasting, incorporating lifestyle practices that nourish the mind, such as regular physical activity, cognitive stimulation, social engagement, and stress management, is essential for promoting cognitive health and vitality.

By cultivating a lifestyle that nurtures both body and mind, we embark upon a journey of cognitive flourishing, imbued with the timeless wisdom of self-care and empowerment.

This chapter illuminates the intricacies of cognitive health and brain aging, offering practical insights into the neuroprotective effects of intermittent fasting for aging women. By embracing mindful lifestyle choices and honoring the profound connection between body and mind, we embark upon a journey of cognitive flourishing, guided by the beacon of holistic well-being.

CHAPTER 7

INFLAMMATION AND IMMUNE FUNCTION

In the intricate dance of health and well-being, inflammation and immune function play pivotal roles, shaping our resilience against illness and fostering vitality. This chapter illuminates the interplay between inflammation and immune function, offering practical insights into reducing inflammation through intermittent fasting and strengthening the immune system in women over 50.

Understanding Inflammation

Inflammation, often hailed as the body's natural response to injury and infection, serves as a double-edged sword. While acute inflammation is a vital component of healing and defense, chronic inflammation can wreak havoc on our health, contributing to a myriad of diseases, including cardiovascular disorders, autoimmune conditions, and metabolic syndrome.

Practical Tips for Reducing Inflammation Through Intermittent Fasting

Intermittent fasting emerges as a promising strategy for taming inflammation and restoring balance to the body's immune response. Here are practical tips for leveraging intermittent fasting to reduce inflammation:

Choose Your Fasting Protocol: Experiment with different fasting protocols, such as time-restricted eating, alternate-day fasting, or periodic fasting, to find the approach that aligns with your lifestyle and health goals.

Focus on Nutrient Density: During eating windows, prioritize nutrient-dense foods rich in antioxidants, anti-inflammatory compounds, and essential nutrients. Incorporate plenty of fruits, vegetables, whole grains, lean proteins, and healthy fats into your meals to support immune function and quell inflammation.

Stay Hydrated: Hydration is key to supporting the body's natural detoxification processes and maintaining optimal immune function. Drink plenty of water throughout the day, and consider incorporating herbal teas and broths during fasting periods to stay hydrated and nourished.

Mindful Movement: Engage in regular physical activity to promote circulation, lymphatic drainage, and overall vitality. Incorporate a mix of cardiovascular exercise, strength training, and flexibility exercises into your routine to support immune function and combat inflammation.

Strengthening the Immune System in Women Over 50

For women over 50, nurturing a robust immune system is essential for maintaining health and vitality. Here are practical tips for strengthening the immune system:

Prioritize Sleep: Quality sleep is essential for immune function and overall well-being. Aim for 7-9 hours of restorative sleep each night, and establish a calming bedtime routine to promote relaxation and optimize sleep quality.

Nutrient-Rich Diet: Embrace a diet rich in immune-boosting nutrients, including vitamin C, vitamin D, zinc, and omega-3 fatty acids. Incorporate a variety of colorful fruits and vegetables, whole grains, lean proteins, and healthy fats into your meals to provide essential nutrients and support immune function.

Manage Stress: Chronic stress can suppress immune function and exacerbate inflammation. Incorporate stress management techniques such as mindfulness meditation, deep breathing exercises, yoga, and time in nature to promote relaxation and resilience.

Stay Active and Social: Engage in regular physical activity and maintain social connections to support immune function and overall well-being. Prioritize activities that bring you joy and foster a sense of community and belonging.

Embracing Wellness Through Inflammation Management and Immune Support

As we navigate the ebbs and flows of health and vitality, embracing strategies to manage inflammation and support immune function becomes paramount. Through the lens of intermittent fasting and holistic lifestyle practices, we empower ourselves to cultivate resilience, vitality, and well-being at every stage of life.

By honoring the innate wisdom of our bodies and nurturing a harmonious balance between inflammation and immune function, we embark upon a journey of holistic wellness, guided by the timeless principles of self-care and empowerment.

This chapter elucidates the intricate relationship between inflammation and immune function, offering practical insights into reducing inflammation through intermittent fasting and strengthening the immune system in women over 50. By embracing mindful lifestyle choices and fostering resilience from within, we embark upon a journey of holistic wellness, fortified by the enduring principles of self-care and empowerment.

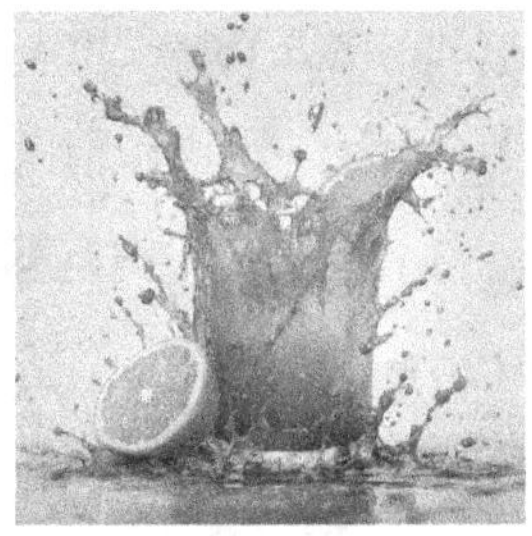

CHAPTER 8

PRACTICAL APPLICATIONS AND GUIDELINES - IMPLEMENTING INTERMITTENT FASTING SAFELY AND EFFECTIVELY

In the realm of health and wellness, intermittent fasting has emerged as a powerful tool for promoting metabolic health, enhancing cellular repair, and fostering longevity. This chapter navigates the practical applications and guidelines for implementing intermittent fasting safely and effectively, drawing upon personal experiences and empirical insights to illuminate the transformative potential of this dietary strategy.

Understanding Intermittent Fasting

A variety of eating schedules that alternate between periods of eating and fasting are included in intermittent fasting. From the popular 16/8 method, which involves fasting for 16 hours and eating within an 8-hour window, to alternate-day fasting and periodic fasting regimens, there exists a spectrum of approaches tailored to individual preferences and goals.

Personal Experience: Navigating the Terrain of Intermittent Fasting

Embarking on my journey of intermittent fasting, I navigated the terrain with a blend of curiosity and caution. Experimenting with different fasting protocols, I discovered insights into hunger cues, metabolic adaptability, and the profound impact of mindful eating practices on overall well-being.

Practical Guidelines for Implementing Intermittent Fasting

Start Gradually: Begin with shorter fasting windows and gradually extend fasting periods as your body adapts. Experiment with different fasting protocols to find the approach that feels sustainable and comfortable for you.

Stay Hydrated: During fasting periods, prioritize hydration by drinking water, herbal teas, and other non-caloric beverages. Staying hydrated supports satiety, promotes detoxification, and mitigates the risk of dehydration during fasting.

Listen to Your Body: Pay attention to hunger cues, energy levels, and overall well-being during fasting periods. Honor your body's signals and be mindful of any adverse effects or discomfort that may arise.

Focus on Nutrient-Dense Foods: When breaking your fast, prioritize nutrient-dense foods rich in vitamins, minerals, and essential nutrients. Incorporate a balance of lean proteins, healthy fats, whole grains, fruits, and vegetables into your meals to support optimal health and satiety.

Mindful Eating Practices: Cultivate mindfulness around food by savoring each bite, chewing slowly, and paying attention to hunger and fullness cues. Mindful eating promotes awareness of dietary choices, fosters a positive relationship with food, and enhances satisfaction during meals.

Tailoring Intermittent Fasting to Individual Needs

When it comes to intermittent fasting, there is no one size fits all solution.. Factors such as age, gender, metabolic health, lifestyle preferences, and underlying medical conditions influence the suitability and efficacy of fasting regimens.

Personalization and Flexibility: Keys to Long-Term Success

Embrace a spirit of personalization and flexibility in your intermittent fasting journey. Listen to your body, adapt your fasting approach as needed, and prioritize overall well-being above rigid adherence to fasting protocols.

Potential Considerations and Precautions

While intermittent fasting offers numerous health benefits, it may not be suitable for everyone. Individuals with certain medical conditions, pregnant or lactating women, and those with a history of disordered eating should exercise caution and consult with a healthcare professional before embarking on an intermittent fasting regimen.

Conclusion: Empowering Health Through Intermittent Fasting

In the tapestry of health and wellness, intermittent fasting emerges as a potent ally, offering a pathway to metabolic health, cellular rejuvenation, and longevity. By embracing practical guidelines, cultivating mindfulness, and honoring the unique needs of our bodies, we empower ourselves to embark upon a journey of holistic well-being, guided by the transformative potential of intermittent fasting.

This chapter navigates the practical applications and guidelines for implementing intermittent fasting safely and effectively, drawing upon personal experiences and empirical insights to illuminate the transformative potential of this dietary strategy. By embracing mindfulness, flexibility, and personalized approaches, we empower ourselves to harness the profound benefits of intermittent fasting on our journey towards optimal health and vitality.

CHAPTER 9

ADDRESSING CONCERNS AND MISCONCEPTIONS

In the landscape of health and wellness, addressing concerns and dispelling misconceptions surrounding fasting and aging is paramount. This chapter delves into common concerns and myths about fasting and aging, drawing upon personal experiences and empirical insights to illuminate the truth behind the veil of uncertainty.

Debunking Myths About Fasting and Aging: A Personal Journey

Embarking on a journey of self-discovery, I encountered a myriad of myths and misconceptions surrounding fasting and aging. From fears of metabolic slowdown to concerns about muscle loss and nutritional deficiencies, the landscape was fraught with uncertainty and apprehension.

Myth 1: Fasting Slows Down Metabolism

One prevailing myth surrounding fasting is that it slows down metabolism, leading to weight gain and metabolic dysfunction. In reality, research suggests that short-term fasting can actually boost metabolic rate by enhancing fat oxidation and promoting metabolic flexibility.

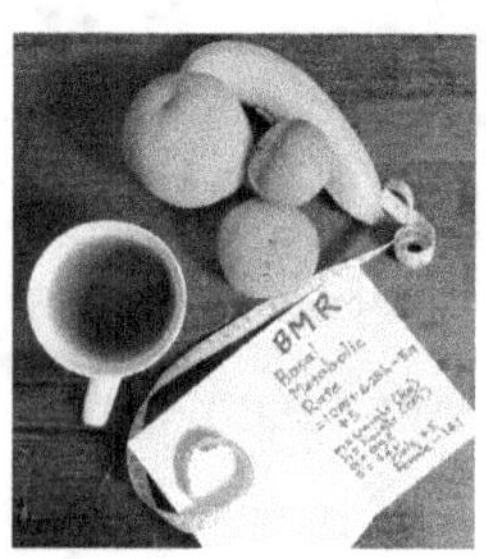

Myth 2: Fasting Causes Muscle Loss

Another common concern is that fasting triggers muscle loss, compromising strength and vitality. While prolonged fasting or severe calorie restriction may indeed lead to muscle breakdown, intermittent fasting has been shown to preserve lean muscle mass and promote fat loss while preserving metabolic health.

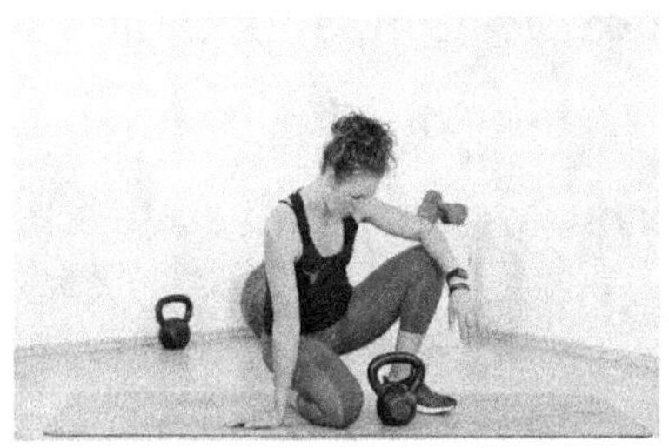

Myth 3: Fasting Leads to Nutritional Deficiencies

Many individuals worry that fasting may result in nutritional deficiencies, depriving the body of essential vitamins, minerals, and nutrients.

However, when approached mindfully and balanced with nutrient-dense eating patterns, intermittent fasting can actually enhance nutrient absorption and support overall well-being.

Addressing Common Concerns: Practical Strategies

Stay Hydrated: Proper hydration is essential during fasting periods to support metabolic function, promote detoxification, and maintain overall well-being. Drink plenty of water, herbal teas, and other non-caloric beverages to stay hydrated and ward off dehydration.

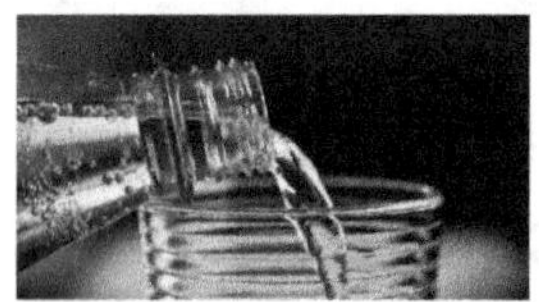

Focus on Nutrient Density: When breaking your fast, prioritize nutrient-dense foods rich in vitamins, minerals, and antioxidants. Incorporate a variety of fruits, vegetables, lean proteins, whole grains, and healthy fats into your meals to support optimal health and vitality.

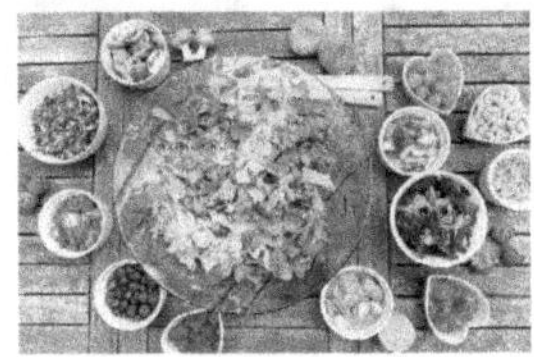

Monitor Energy Levels: Pay attention to your body's signals and adjust your fasting approach accordingly. If you experience fatigue, dizziness, or other adverse effects, consider modifying your fasting protocol or seeking guidance from a healthcare professional.

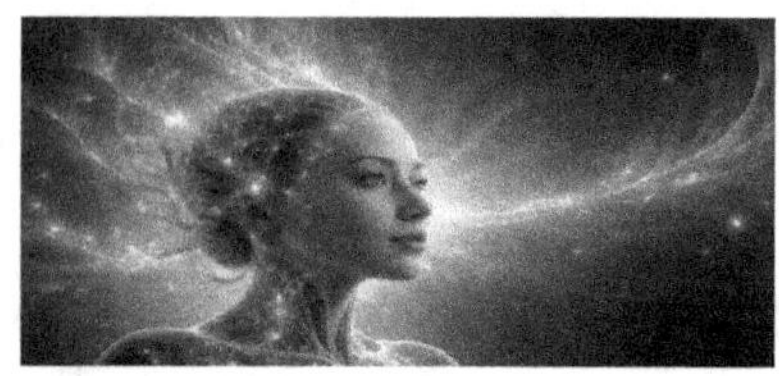

Embrace Flexibility: Remember that intermittent fasting is not a one-size-fits-all approach. Tailor your fasting regimen to suit your individual needs, preferences, and lifestyle constraints. Experiment with different fasting protocols and find the approach that works best for you.

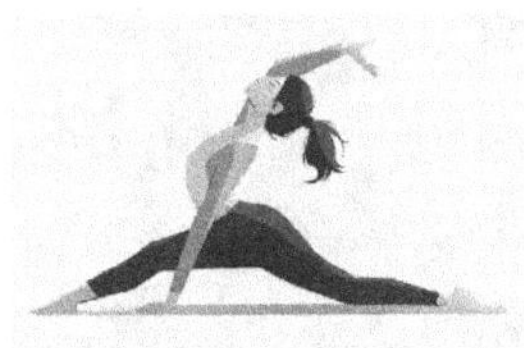

Navigating the Journey of Fasting and Aging

In the tapestry of health and aging, navigating the terrain of fasting requires a blend of curiosity, mindfulness, and discernment. By dispelling myths, addressing concerns, and embracing evidence-based practices, we empower ourselves to embark upon a journey of holistic well-being, guided by the wisdom of self-discovery and empowerment.

Conclusion: Embracing Truth and Empowerment

As we unravel the tapestry of myths and misconceptions surrounding fasting and aging, let us embrace the truth with courage and clarity. By fostering a spirit of inquiry, openness, and discernment, we empower ourselves to transcend limitations, embrace possibilities, and embark upon a journey of vibrant health and vitality.

CHAPTER 10

RECIPES AND SPICES THAT CAN HELP WOMEN OVER 50 REGAIN THEIR HEALTH WHILE PRACTICING INTERMITTENT FASTING.

Here are recipes across various categories to help women over 50 regain their health while practicing intermittent fasting:

Breakfast

Greek Yogurt Parfait: Layer Greek yogurt with mixed berries and a sprinkle of almonds or walnuts. Serve with a drizzle of honey or a dash of cinnamon.

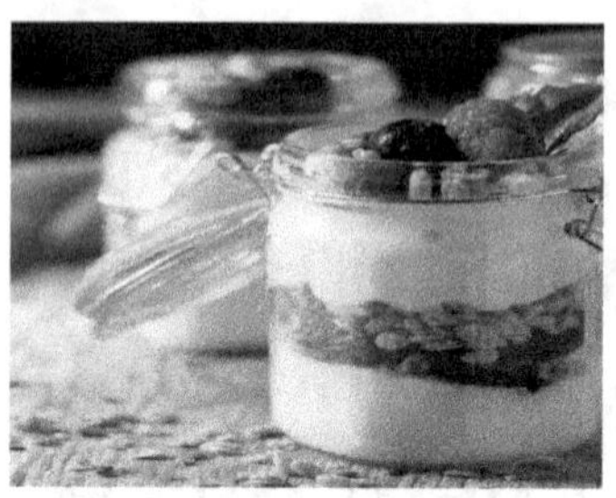

Avocado Toast: Top whole grain toast with mashed avocado, sliced tomatoes, and a poached egg. For seasoning, add a little lemon juice, salt, and pepper.

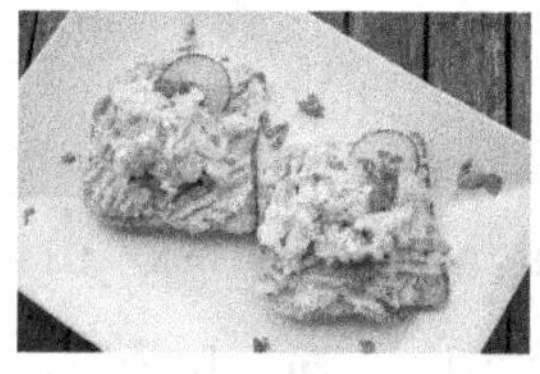

Coconut Chia Seed Pudding: Mix chia seeds with coconut milk, a splash of vanilla extract, and a pinch of cinnamon. Let it sit in the refrigerator overnight and top with toasted coconut flakes and sliced tropical fruits in the morning.

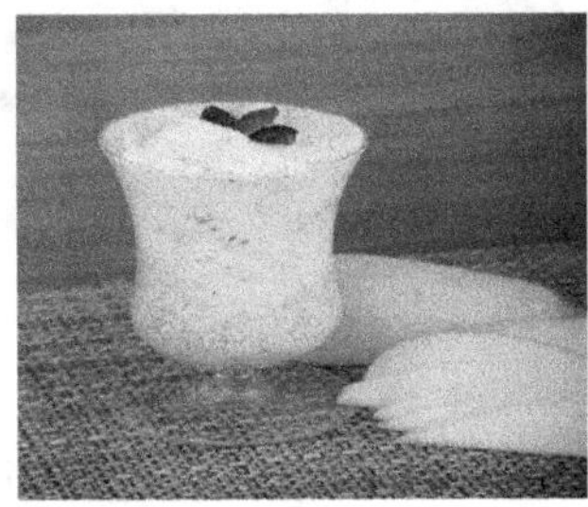

Sesame Ginger Tofu Bowl: Marinate cubed tofu in a mixture of sesame oil, soy sauce, ginger, and garlic. Sauté until golden brown and serve over brown rice or quinoa with steamed broccoli and a sprinkle of sesame seeds.

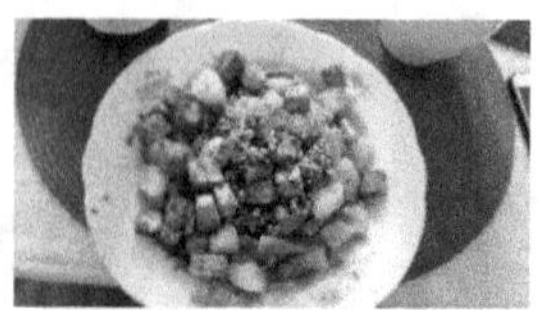

Tofu Scramble Breakfast Tacos: Sauté crumbled tofu with bell peppers, onions, and spinach. Serve in whole grain tortillas topped with salsa, avocado slices, and a sprinkle of nutritional yeast for a savory morning meal.

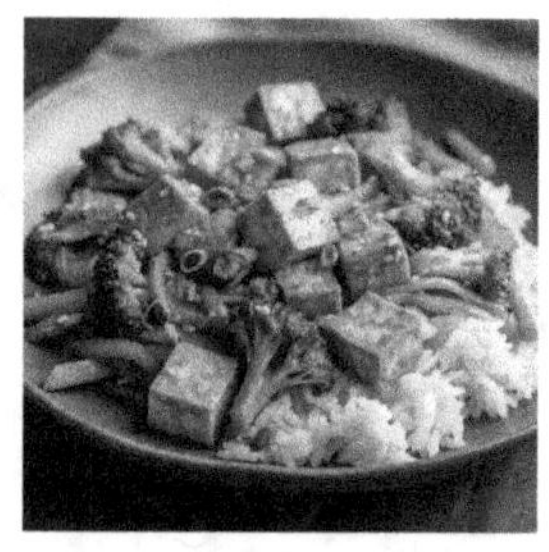

Green Smoothie Bowl: Blend spinach, kale, banana, avocado, and almond milk until smooth. Pour into a bowl and top with granola, sliced kiwi, and a sprinkle of hemp seeds for a nutrient-packed start to the day.

Lunch

Quinoa Salad: Toss cooked quinoa with mixed greens, diced cucumber, cherry tomatoes, avocado slices, and grilled chicken or tofu. Dress with a lemon vinaigrette.

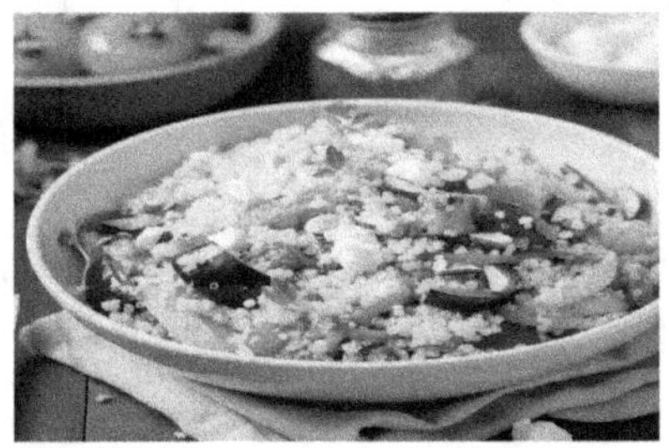

Mediterranean Chickpea Salad: Combine chickpeas with chopped cucumber, bell peppers, red onion, Kalamata olives, and feta cheese. Add oregano, lemon juice, and olive oil as dressings.

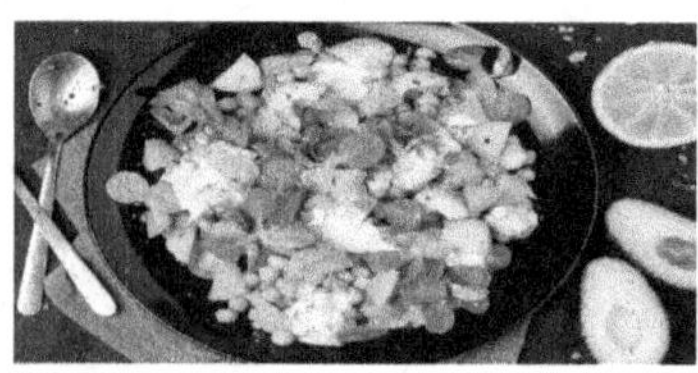

Soba Noodle Salad with Miso Dressing: Toss cooked soba noodles with shredded cabbage, edamame, shredded carrots, and sliced cucumbers. Drizzle with a homemade miso dressing made with miso paste, rice vinegar, sesame oil, and a touch of honey.

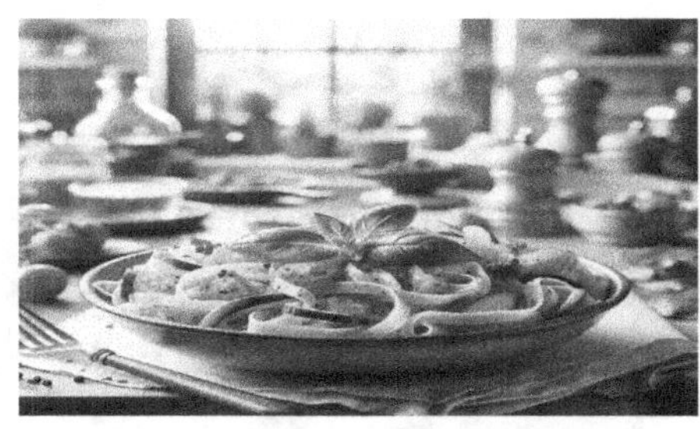

Mango Chicken Lettuce Wraps: Fill lettuce leaves with diced cooked chicken, fresh mango cubes, avocado slices, and a squeeze of lime juice. Sprinkle with chopped cilantro and a drizzle of tahini sauce.

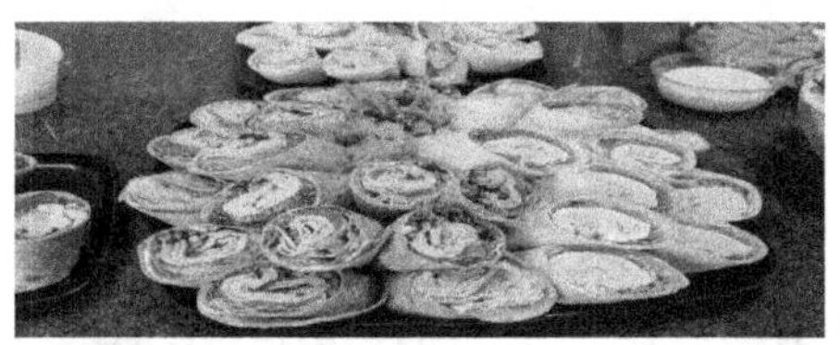

Salmon and Avocado Nori Wraps: Spread mashed avocado on sheets of nori and top with flaked cooked salmon, cucumber strips, and shredded carrots. Roll tightly and slice into sushi-style pieces for a refreshing and satisfying lunch.

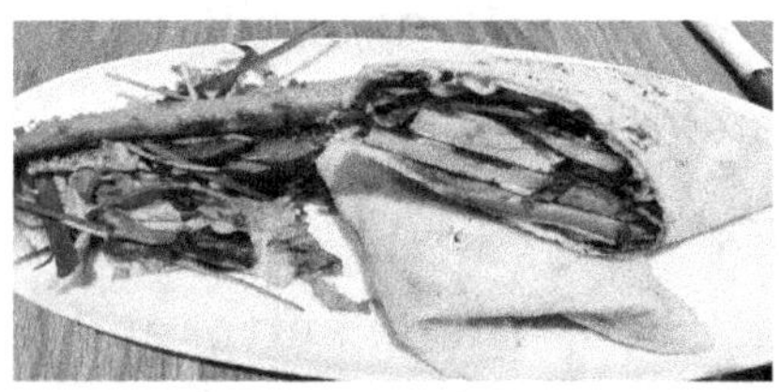

Dinner

Garlic, dill, and lemon zest: are used to season salmon fillets for grilled salmon with asparagus. Grill until cooked through and serve with roasted asparagus spears.

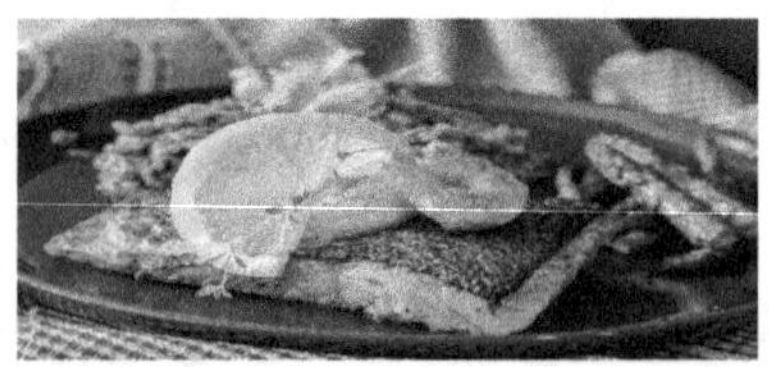

Turkey and Vegetable Stir-Fry: Stir-fry lean turkey strips with bell peppers, snap peas, carrots, and broccoli in a light soy sauce. Serve over cauliflower rice.

Pesto-Spiraled Zucchini Noodles: Prepare a homemade or store-bought pesto sauce and toss with the noodles. Top with grilled shrimp or roasted cherry tomatoes for added flavor.

Cauliflower Crust Pizza: Make a pizza crust using cauliflower rice, almond flour, eggs, and Italian seasoning. Top with marinara sauce, mozzarella cheese, and your favorite vegetables before baking until golden and crispy.

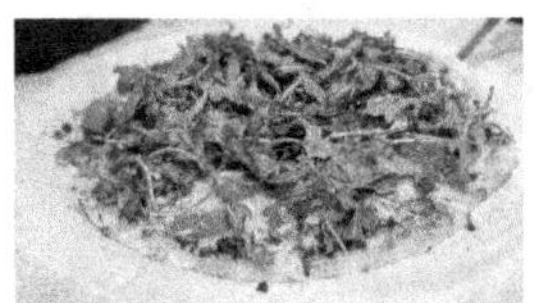

Stuffed Bell Peppers: Stuff cooked quinoa, black beans, corn, diced tomatoes, and spices inside of half bell peppers. Top with shredded cheese and bake until peppers are tender and filling is heated through.

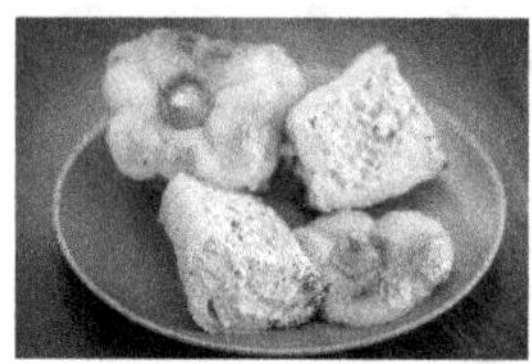

Cauliflower Fried Rice: Pulse cauliflower florets in a food processor until rice-like in texture. Sauté with diced vegetables, scrambled eggs, and cooked shrimp or tofu in a wok with soy sauce and sesame oil for a low-carb twist on a classic dish.

Snacks

Almond Butter Apple Slices: Spread almond butter on apple slices and sprinkle with chia seeds or granola for added crunch.

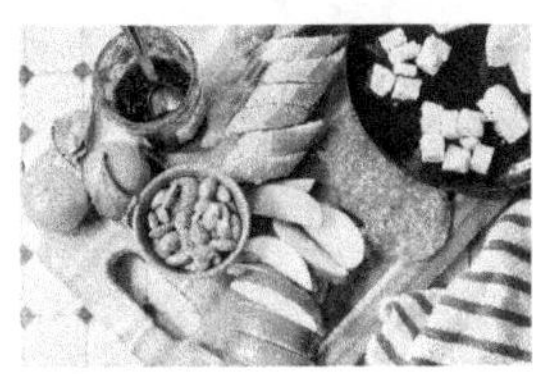

Greek Yogurt with Berries: Top a serving of Greek yogurt with fresh berries and a drizzle of honey or a sprinkle of granola.

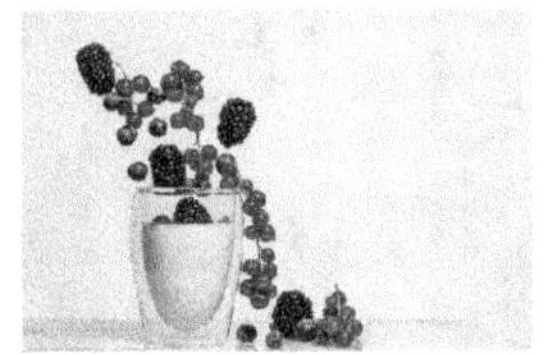

Turmeric Roasted Chickpeas: Toss cooked chickpeas with olive oil, turmeric, cumin, and a pinch of sea salt. Roast in the oven until crispy for a flavorful and satisfying snack.

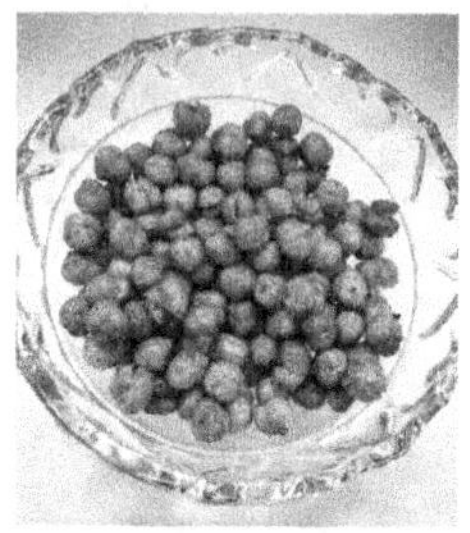

Edamame Hummus: Blend cooked edamame with tahini, lemon juice, garlic, and a touch of olive oil until smooth. Serve with whole grain crackers for dipping or with sliced vegetables.

Turmeric Roasted Cauliflower Bites: Toss cauliflower florets with olive oil, turmeric, smoked paprika, and a pinch of salt. Roast in the oven until golden brown and crispy for a flavorful and nutritious snack.

Desserts

Chia Seed Pudding: Mix chia seeds with almond milk, vanilla extract, and a touch of maple syrup. Let sit overnight in the refrigerator and top with fresh fruit before serving.

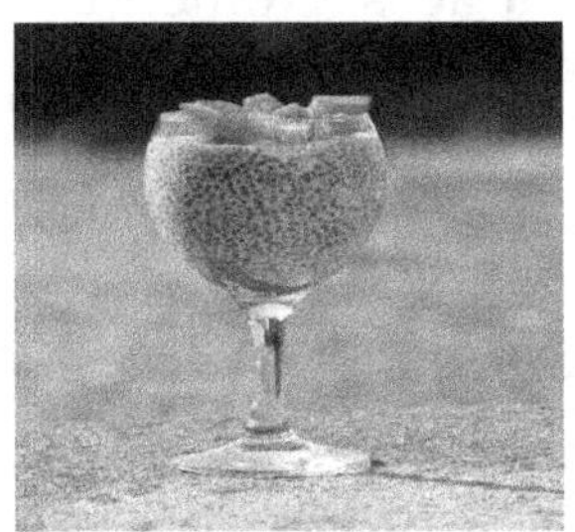

Dark Chocolate Bark: Melt dark chocolate and spread it on a baking sheet lined with parchment paper. Sprinkle with nuts, seeds, and dried fruit. Allow to harden in the refrigerator before breaking into pieces.

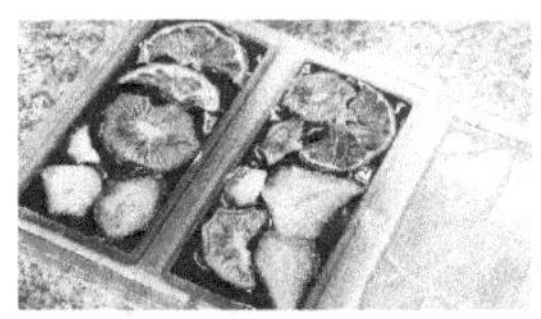

These recipes are designed to provide nutrient-rich, balanced meals that support overall health and well-being while aligning with intermittent fasting practices. Remember to adjust portion sizes and meal timings according to individual fasting schedules and dietary preferences.

Berry Coconut Bliss Balls: Blend dried mixed berries, shredded coconut, almond flour, and a drizzle of honey in a food processor until a dough forms. Form into little balls and place in the refrigerator to solidify.

Egg Muffins: Whisk together eggs, diced vegetables, and cooked turkey sausage or bacon. Pour into muffin tins and bake until set for a convenient and portable breakfast option.

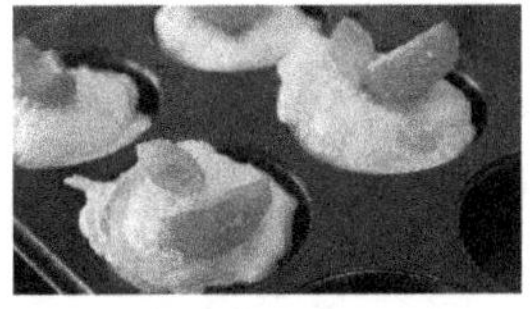

Roasted Beet Hummus: Blend roasted beets with chickpeas, lemon juice, garlic, and a drizzle of olive oil until smooth. Serve with carrot sticks, cucumber slices, or whole grain crackers for dipping.

Frozen Banana Bites: Dip banana slices in melted dark chocolate and sprinkle with chopped nuts or coconut flakes. Place on a parchment-lined tray and freeze until set for a guilt-free sweet treat.

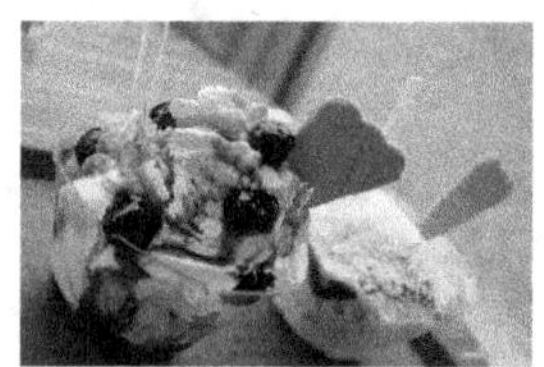

Chia Seed Chocolate Pudding: Blend chia seeds with unsweetened almond milk, cocoa powder, a touch of maple syrup, and a dash of vanilla extract. Let it sit in the refrigerator until thickened and top with fresh berries before serving.

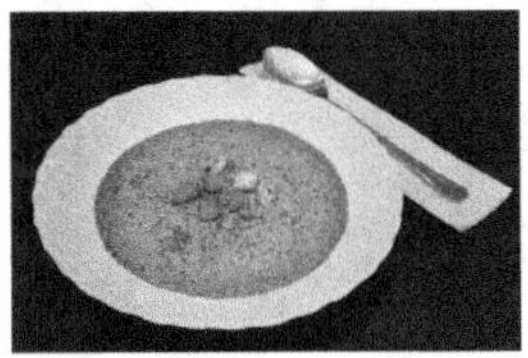

Coconut Matcha Chia Pudding: Mix chia seeds with coconut milk, matcha powder, and a touch of honey. Let it sit in the refrigerator until thickened and top with toasted coconut flakes for a refreshing and energizing dessert option.

Here are healthy spices that can enhance overall health and contribute to a vibrant appearance for women over 50 practicing intermittent fasting:

Turmeric: Known for its potent anti-inflammatory properties, turmeric contains curcumin, which helps reduce inflammation, support joint health, and promote radiant skin.

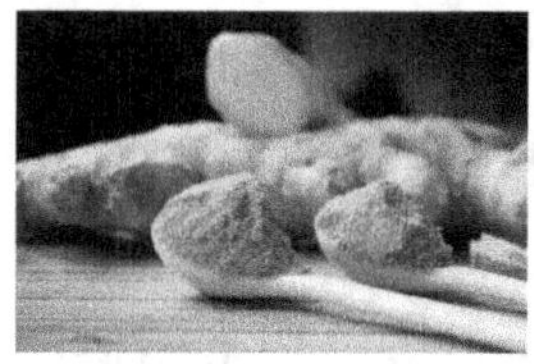

Cinnamon: This versatile spice not only adds flavor but also helps regulate blood sugar levels, improve insulin sensitivity, and enhance metabolism, making it beneficial for weight management and overall health.

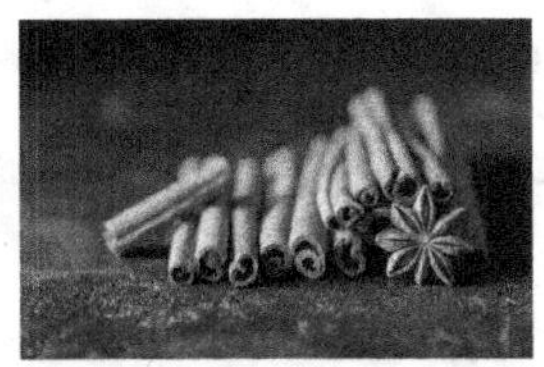

Ginger: With its warming and invigorating qualities, ginger aids digestion, reduces inflammation, and supports immune function. It can also help alleviate nausea and promote healthy circulation.

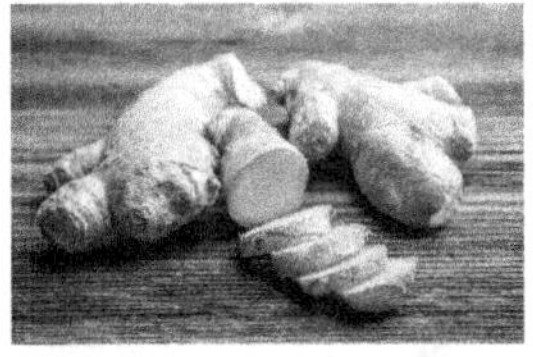

Cayenne Pepper: Rich in capsaicin, cayenne pepper has thermogenic properties that can boost metabolism, promote fat burning, and suppress appetite, making it an excellent addition to weight management efforts.

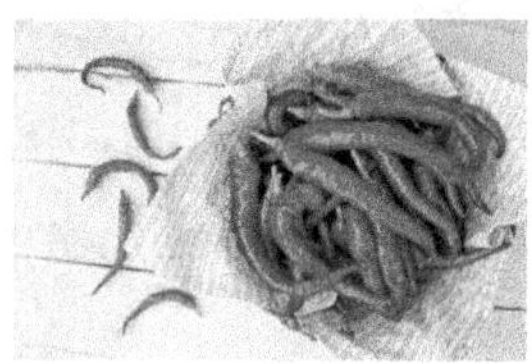

Garlic: Besides adding flavor to dishes, garlic offers numerous health benefits, including cardiovascular support, immune enhancement, and antimicrobial properties that can help combat infections and promote gut health.

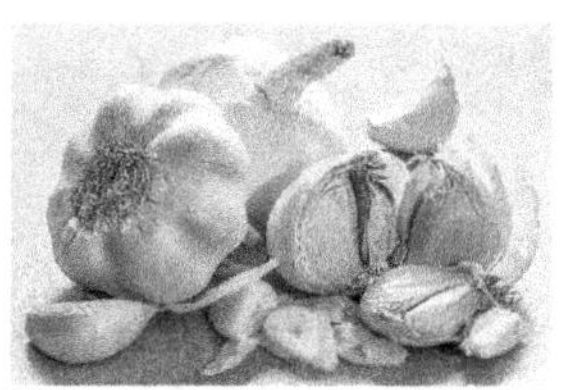

Cumin: This aromatic spice is rich in antioxidants and may help improve digestion, reduce bloating, and alleviate symptoms of irritable bowel syndrome (IBS), supporting gastrointestinal health and overall well-being.

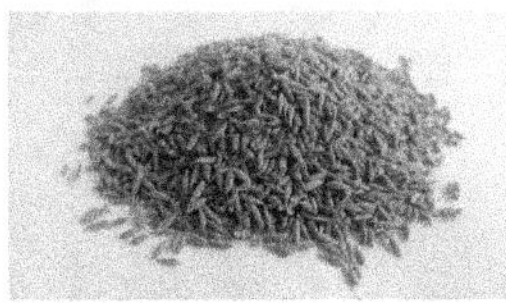

Cardamom: With its unique flavor and aroma, cardamom is not only delicious but also offers digestive support, helps regulate blood sugar levels, and may have antimicrobial properties that support oral health.

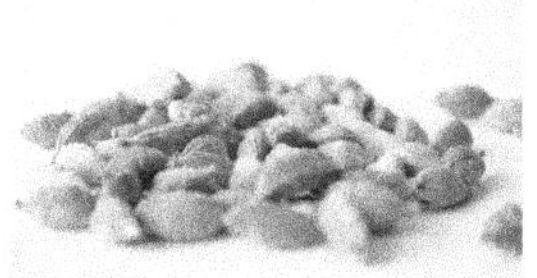

Black Pepper: In addition to enhancing the taste of food, black pepper contains piperine, a compound that can enhance nutrient absorption, improve digestion, and potentially aid in weight management.

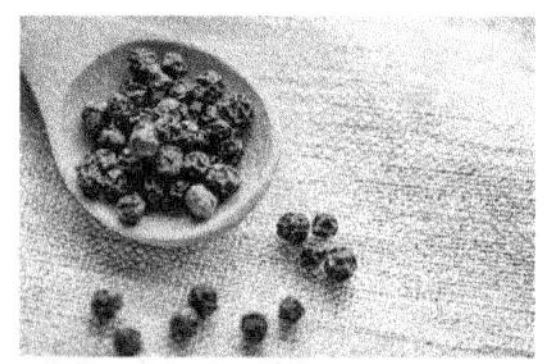

Rosemary: This fragrant herb contains antioxidants and anti-inflammatory compounds that may help protect against oxidative stress, support cognitive function, and promote healthy aging.

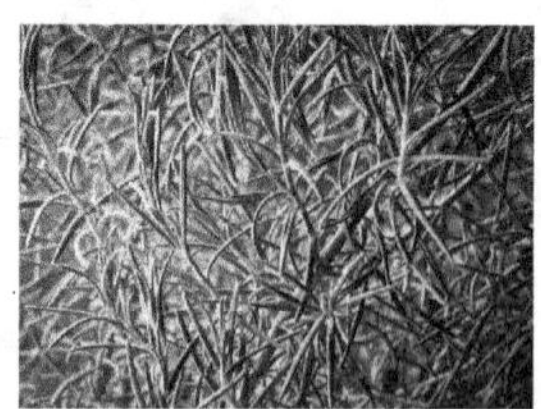

Saffron: Known for its distinct flavor and vibrant color, saffron contains compounds that have been shown to have antidepressant effects, support mood regulation, and improve cognitive function.

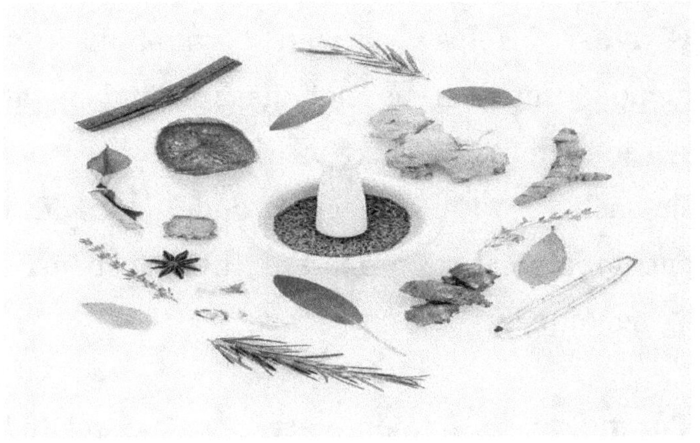

For women over 50, incorporating spices into their diet can offer a range of health benefits tailored to their specific needs:

Ginger: Helps alleviate symptoms of menopause such as hot flashes and night sweats, supports digestion which may become sluggish with age, and provides anti-inflammatory properties that can benefit aging joints.

Turmeric: Counteracts age-related inflammation, supports joint health, and may help maintain cognitive function, which is especially important as women age and face increased risk of conditions like Alzheimer's disease.

Cinnamon: Supports blood sugar regulation, which becomes more challenging with age and can help prevent age-related insulin resistance and type 2 diabetes.

Cayenne pepper: Boosts metabolism, which tends to slow down with age, and may aid in weight management, which can become more challenging post-menopause due to hormonal changes.

Garlic: Supports heart health by lowering cholesterol and blood pressure levels, which are important considerations for women over 50 who may be at increased risk of heart disease.

Cumin: Aids digestion and nutrient absorption, which can become less efficient with age, and may also help regulate blood sugar levels and support weight management.

Cardamom: Supports digestive health, which may become more sensitive with age, and provides antioxidant properties that help combat age-related oxidative stress.

Black pepper: Enhances nutrient absorption, which becomes more important as nutrient needs may increase with age, and supports digestive function to alleviate age-related digestive issues.

Rosemary: Supports cognitive function and memory, which may decline with age, and provides antioxidant properties that help protect against age-related cognitive decline and neurodegenerative diseases.

Saffron: Helps regulate mood and reduce stress, which can become more prevalent with age, and provides antioxidant properties that help protect against age-related oxidative damage.

By incorporating these spices into their diet, women over 50 can support their overall health and well-being as they navigate the unique challenges and considerations of aging.

CHAPTER 11

PERSONAL STORIES AND TESTIMONIALS

In the realm of intermittent fasting, personal stories and testimonials serve as beacons of inspiration, offering insights and motivation for individuals embarking on their own fasting journeys. This chapter illuminates the real-life experiences of women over 50 who practice intermittent fasting, drawing upon personal anecdotes, insights, and inspiration to empower readers on their path to wellness and vitality.

Real-Life Experiences of Women Over 50 Who Practice Intermittent Fasting

Jane's Journey: Embracing Empowerment Through Fasting

For Jane, a vibrant woman in her 50s, intermittent fasting became a catalyst for transformation and empowerment. Struggling with weight management and fluctuating energy levels, Jane turned to intermittent fasting as a sustainable approach to reclaiming her health and vitality.

"Jane remembers, "I was sick of rigid diets and never-ending cycles of weight loss and gain. "Intermittent fasting offered me a new perspective—a way to nourish my body, balance my hormones, and embrace a lifestyle of empowerment."

Through mindful fasting protocols and a commitment to self-care, Jane discovered newfound energy, mental clarity, and a renewed sense of vitality. By honoring her body's innate wisdom and fostering a positive relationship with food, Jane embarked on a journey of holistic well-being that transcended mere physical transformation.

Susan's Story: Finding Freedom and Flexibility Through Fasting

Susan, a dynamic woman in her 60s, found liberation and flexibility in the practice of intermittent fasting. Juggling a busy career, family responsibilities, and a desire for optimal health, Susan sought a sustainable approach to nourishing her body and nurturing her spirit.

"I was able to enjoy food guilt-free and without limitations thanks to intermittent fasting," Susan muses. "I no longer felt enslaved by the clock or the tyranny of constant snacking.

Fasting allowed me to savor each meal, cultivate mindfulness, and reclaim my time and energy."

Through trial and error, Susan discovered the fasting protocols that resonated with her lifestyle and goals. By embracing flexibility, adapting to her body's changing needs, and prioritizing self-care, Susan forged a path of wellness that celebrated balance, abundance, and joy.

Insights and Inspiration from Successful Fasters

Mindful Eating Practices

Many successful fasters emphasize the importance of mindful eating practices. By savoring each bite, chewing slowly, and paying attention to hunger and fullness cues, individuals can cultivate a deeper connection with food and foster a positive relationship with eating.

Adaptability and Flexibility

Successful fasters recognize the value of adaptability and flexibility in their fasting journeys. Rather than adhering rigidly to preset protocols, they listen to their bodies, adjust their fasting approach as needed, and prioritize overall well-being above strict adherence to rules.

Community and Support

Building a supportive community of fellow fasters can provide invaluable encouragement, accountability, and camaraderie. Sharing experiences, exchanging tips, and celebrating milestones together can foster a sense of belonging and empowerment on the fasting journey.

Self-Compassion and Resilience

Embracing self-compassion and resilience is essential for navigating the ups and downs of intermittent fasting. Recognizing that setbacks and challenges are natural parts of the journey, successful fasters approach setbacks with kindness, patience, and a steadfast commitment to growth and self-discovery.Embracing the Journey of Intermittent Fasting

In the tapestry of wellness and vitality, personal stories and testimonials serve as powerful reminders of the transformative potential of intermittent fasting. Through the lens of real-life experiences, women over 50 find empowerment, inspiration, and renewal on their fasting journeys.

As we embark upon the path of intermittent fasting, let us embrace the wisdom of those who have gone before us, drawing upon their insights, resilience, and courage to forge our own paths of wellness and vitality. By honoring the unique journey of each individual and celebrating the collective power of shared experiences, we pave the way for a future of holistic health and vibrant living.

This chapter illuminates the real-life experiences of women over 50 who practice intermittent fasting, drawing upon personal anecdotes, insights, and inspiration to empower readers on their path to wellness and vitality. Through stories of empowerment, freedom, and resilience, women find renewal and inspiration to embrace the transformative potential of intermittent fasting in their own lives.

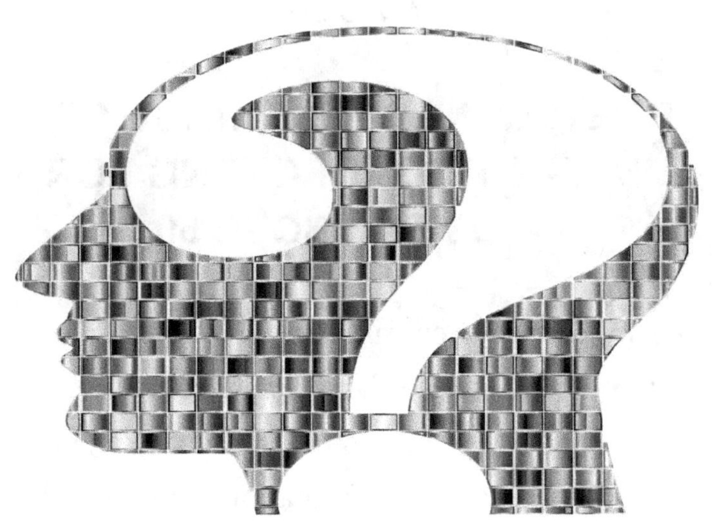

CONCLUSION

EMBRACING THE JOURNEY OF INTERMITTENT FASTING FOR WOMEN ABOVE 50

As we draw the curtains on our exploration of intermittent fasting for women above 50, we embark upon a journey of reflection, inspiration, and transformation. Through the tapestry of personal stories, scientific insights, and practical wisdom, we have unearthed the timeless principles of longevity and aging gracefully, guided by the transformative potential of intermittent fasting.

In the realm of wellness and vitality, intermittent fasting emerges as a beacon of hope, offering a pathway to holistic health, resilience, and vitality. From the bustling streets of metabolic rejuvenation to the tranquil shores of cellular repair, the journey of intermittent fasting beckons us to embrace the boundless possibilities of our own potential.

Embracing the Wisdom of Aging Gracefully

At its core, intermittent fasting invites us to embrace the wisdom of aging gracefully—to honor the sacred covenant between body, mind, and spirit, and to nurture the flame of vitality that burns brightly within. Through mindful fasting protocols, nourishing dietary choices, and a commitment to holistic well-being, we unlock the secret to longevity, vitality, and radiant health.

Navigating the Terrain of Intermittent Fasting

Along the journey of intermittent fasting, we encounter moments of triumph and challenge, growth and transformation. We learn to listen to the whispers of our bodies, to heed the call of intuition, and to embrace the rhythm of life with grace and resilience.

Through the prism of intermittent fasting, we discover the power of adaptation and flexibility—the ability to pivot, to evolve, and to thrive in the face of uncertainty. We recognize that the journey is not one of perfection, but of progress—a tapestry woven with threads of courage, perseverance, and self-discovery.

Cultivating Resilience and Vitality

As women above 50, we stand at the threshold of possibility, poised to embark upon a journey of renewal and vitality. With each passing day, we embrace the wisdom of experience, the beauty of imperfection, and the profound gift of self-awareness.

Through the gentle cadence of intermittent fasting, we nurture the flame of resilience within us—a flame that flickers with the promise of renewal, the joy of discovery, and the grace of acceptance. We honor the ebb and flow of life, the rhythm of seasons, and the immutable passage of time with gratitude and reverence.

Embracing the Central Message of Intermittent Fasting

As we reflect upon the central message of intermittent fasting for women above 50, we are reminded of its timeless wisdom—a wisdom that transcends the boundaries of age, gender, and circumstance. It is a wisdom that speaks to the essence of our humanity, the resilience of our spirit, and the infinite potential that resides within each of us.

Intermittent fasting invites us to reclaim our vitality, to honor our bodies as temples of wisdom, and to embrace the journey of aging with grace and dignity. It is a journey that invites us to awaken to the beauty of the present moment, to savor the richness of life, and to celebrate the miracle of our own existence.

A Call to Action: Embrace the Journey

As we bid farewell to these pages, let us carry forth the flame of inspiration, the torch of wisdom, and the spirit of resilience into our daily lives. Let us embrace the journey of intermittent fasting with courage and conviction, knowing that each step we take brings us closer to the radiant vitality that awaits us.

Let us nourish our bodies with love and reverence, cultivate our minds with curiosity and wonder, and nurture our spirits with grace and compassion. Let us stand as beacons of hope, guardians of wellness, and champions of vitality for ourselves and for generations to come.

In Closing: A Future of Possibility

In closing, let us envision a future of possibility—a future where women over 50 embrace the transformative power of intermittent fasting, where vitality knows no bounds, and where the journey of aging is celebrated as a testament to the resilience of the human spirit.

May we walk this path with grace and dignity, with courage and conviction, knowing that the journey of intermittent fasting is not just a destination, but a sacred pilgrimage—a journey of self-discovery, empowerment, and boundless potential.

As we turn the page to a new chapter, may we carry the wisdom of intermittent fasting in our hearts, the light of inspiration in our souls, and the promise of vitality in our spirits. For in the journey of aging gracefully lies the infinite possibility of a life well-lived—a life imbued with purpose, passion, and radiant vitality.

As we bid farewell to the journey of intermittent fasting for women above 50, let us embrace the wisdom, inspiration, and transformation it has bestowed upon us. With courage and conviction, let us embark upon a future of possibility, where the flame of vitality burns brightly within us, guiding us towards a life of resilience, wellness, and fulfillment.

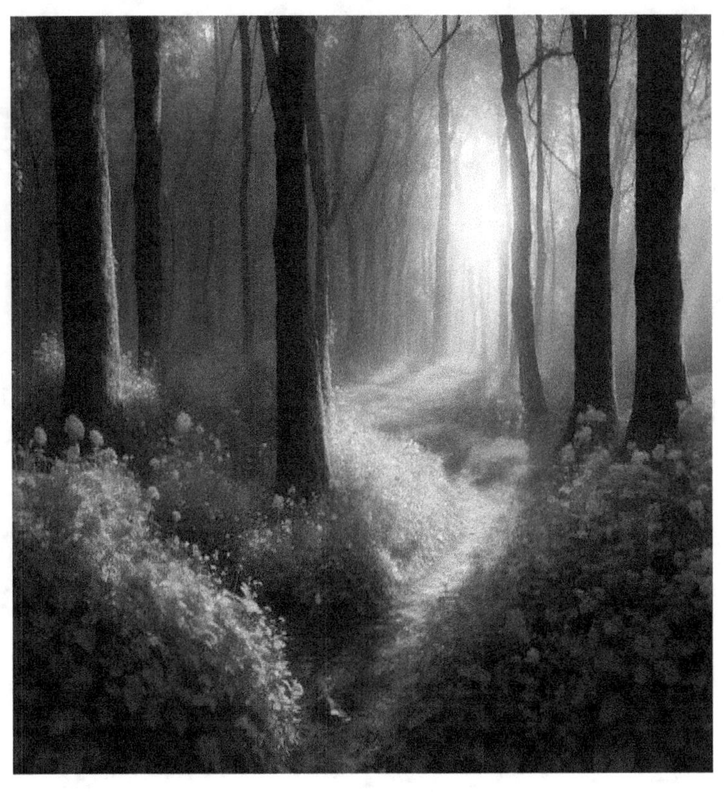

www.ingramcontent.com/pod-product-compliance
Lightning Source LLC
Chambersburg PA
CBHW061653250726

48659CB00004B/1483